25 Delicious Recipes for Healthier and Younger Skin

Disclaimer and Terms of Use:

Effort has been made to ensure that the information in this book is accurate and complete, however, the author and the publisher do not warrant the accuracy of the information, text and graphics contained within the book due to the rapidly changing nature of science, research, known and unknown facts and internet. The Author and the publisher do not hold any responsibility for errors, omissions or contrary interpretation of the subject matter herein. This book is presented solely for motivational and informational purposes only.

Table of Contents

Introduction

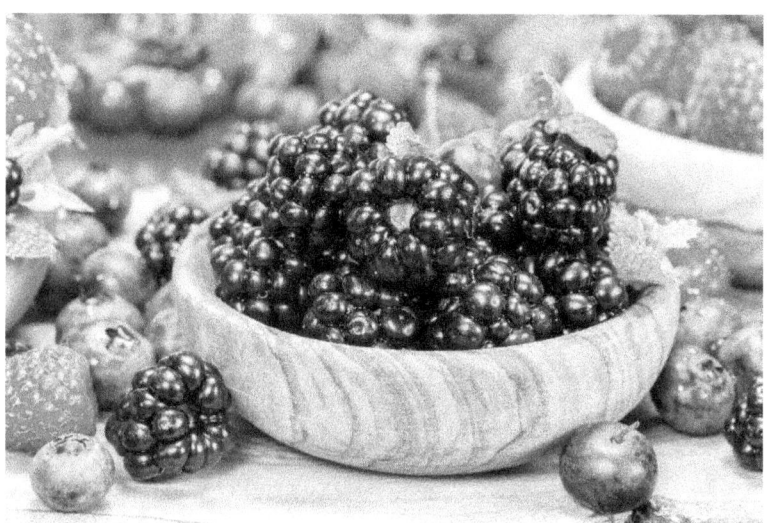

Subjecting your body to invasive surgeries can cost you a fortune or even your beauty. If you're trying to look younger and don't want to go through surgery, then you're going to be glad you found this book. This book will give you twenty-five delicious recipes and may be changing your diet, so you can have younger looking skin. Nourishing your insides affects the way your skin glows. You can easily remove years on your skin and face just by making changed to the food that you eat. If you add an exercise routine to this diet, you can boost the results of the anti-aging effects these recipes will give you. So what are you waiting for? Come and indulge yourself in great, delicious food that feeds not only you but also your mind and body.

Banana High-Protein Smoothie

Servings: 1

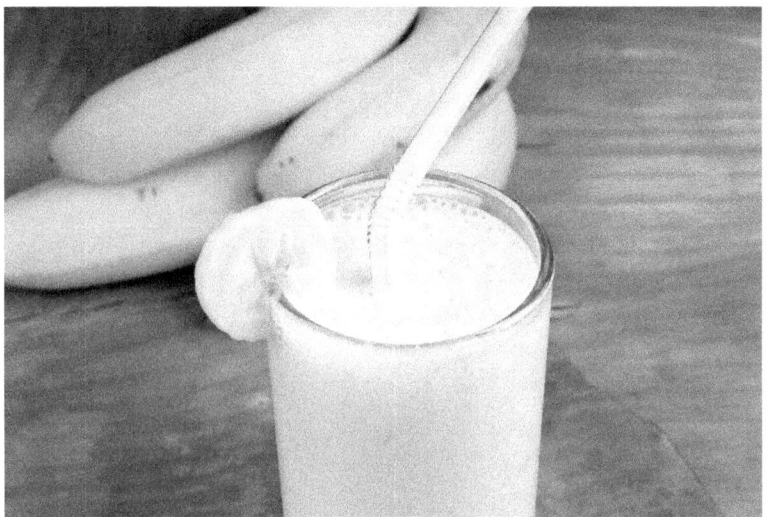

Ingredients:

1 cup plain Greek yogurt

1 large frozen banana, peeled and sliced

1 scoop vanilla protein powder

½ cup skim milk

2 tablespoons peanut butter

Instructions:

1. In a blender, add all of the ingredients.
2. Blend until smooth, about 30 to 60 seconds.
3. Pour in a glass and enjoy.

Blueberry Smoothie

Servings: 1

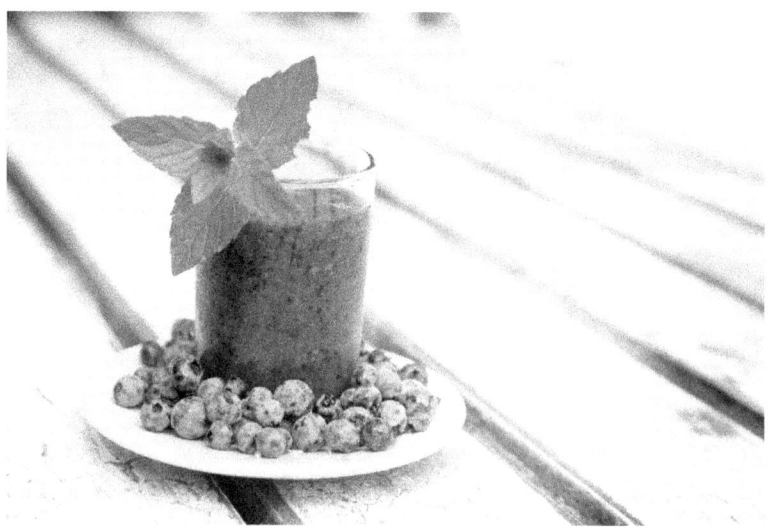

Ingredients:

1 ½ cups frozen blueberries

1 cup skim milk

½ cup plain Greek yogurt

5 to 6 ice cubes

2 tablespoons fresh chopped mint

Instructions:

1. Add all of the ingredients in a blender.
2. Blend until smooth and combined.
3. Pour in a glass and enjoy cold.

Chocolate Protein Smoothie

Servings: 1

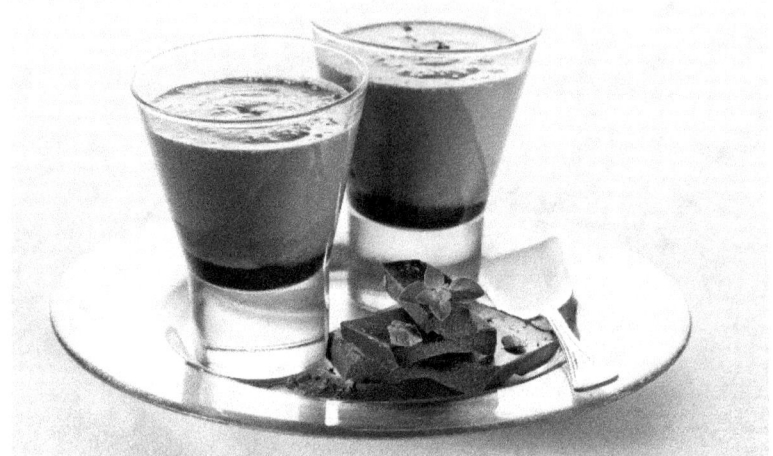

Ingredients:

1 cup chocolate soy milk

1 large frozen banana, peeled and sliced

1 scoop chocolate protein powder

½ cup plain Greek yogurt

2 tablespoons chia seeds

Instructions:

1. In a blender, add all of the ingredients.
2. Blend until smooth, about 30 to 60 seconds.
3. Pour in a glass and enjoy.

Blackberry Yogurt Smoothie

Servings: 1

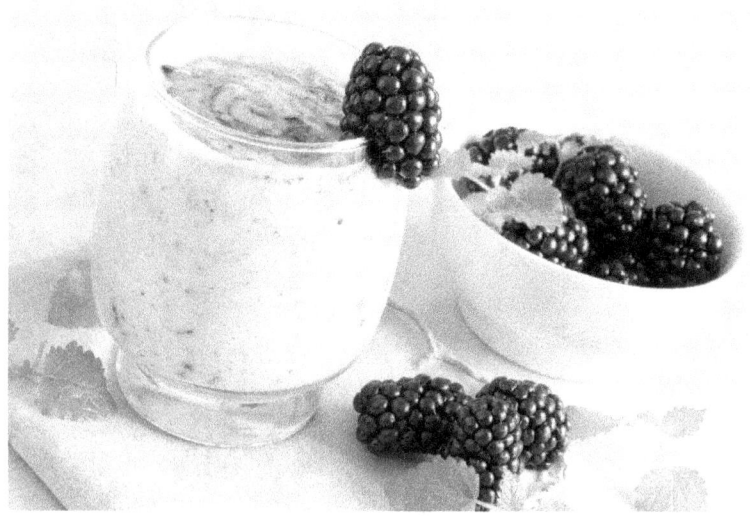

Ingredients:

1 ½ cups frozen blackberries

1 cup plain Greek yogurt

1 scoop vanilla protein powder

1 teaspoon honey

½ cup skim milk

Instructions:

1. In a blender, add all of the ingredients.
2. Blend until smooth, about 30 to 60 seconds.
3. Pour in a glass and enjoy.

Tropical Smoothie

Servings: 1

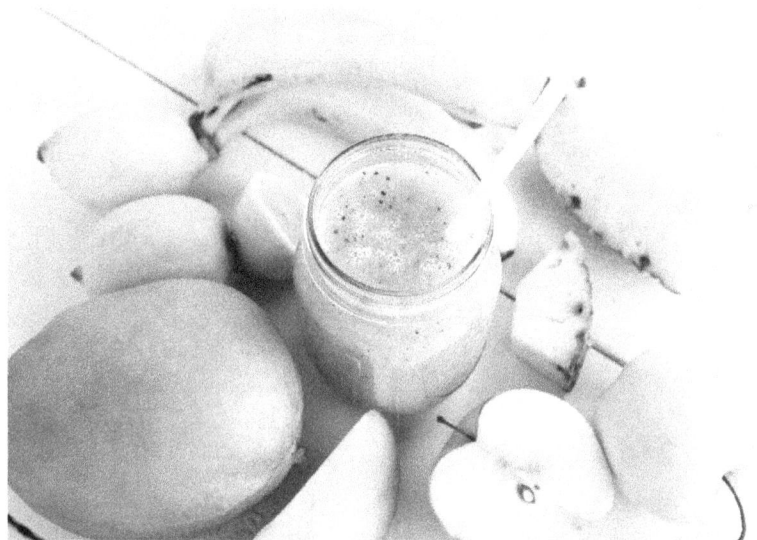

Ingredients:

1 cup frozen pineapple chunks

1 cup skim milk

1 small frozen banana, peeled and sliced

½ cup frozen mango chunks

½ cup plain Greek yogurt

Instructions:

1. In a high-speed blender, add all the ingredients.
2. Blend for about 30 to 60 seconds on high until smooth.

3. Pour in a glass and enjoy.

Sweet Grape Smoothie

Servings: 1

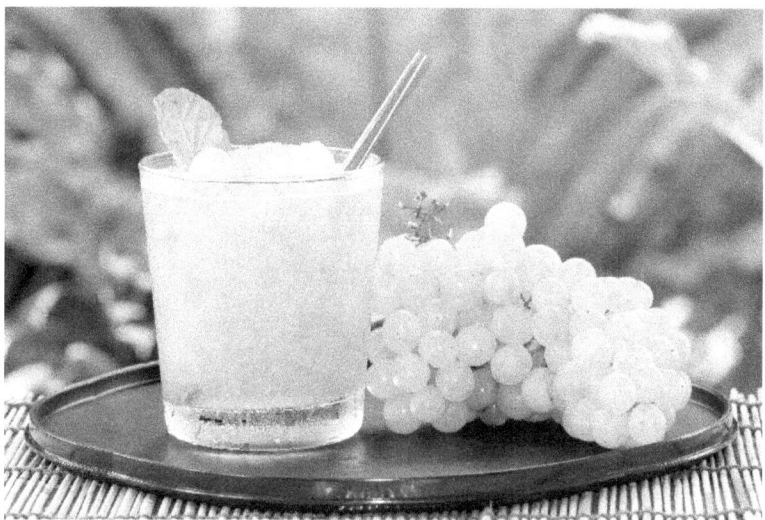

Ingredients:

1 cup seedless green grapes

1 large frozen banana, peeled and sliced

½ cup fresh orange juice

¼ cup plain Greek yogurt

Instructions:

1. In a blender, add all of the ingredients.
2. Blend for about 30 to 60 seconds on high or until smooth.
3. Pour in a glass and enjoy.

Eggs Baked in Avocado

Servings: 6

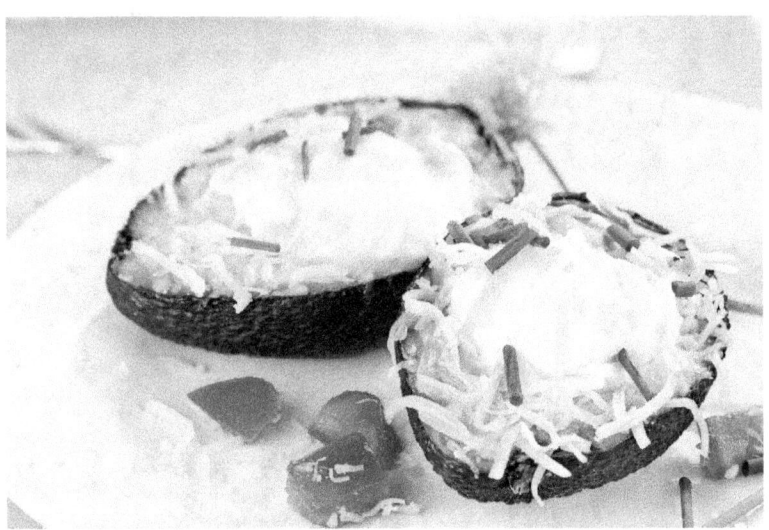

Ingredients:

½ cup shredded cheddar cheese

¼ cup fresh chopped chives

3 medium ripe avocado

6 large eggs

Salt and pepper to taste

Instructions:

1. Preheat the oven to 425°F/220°C.
2. Cut the avocados lengthwise and remove the pits.
3. Place the avocados in a oven safe glass baking dish.

4. Remove about 2 tablespoons of the avocado flesh from each of the halves.
5. Crack one egg in each of the halves and season with salt and pepper.
6. Sprinkle with cheese and chives on top of the egg.
7. Bake for about 15 to 20 minutes or until the egg is cooked as desired.

Refreshing Fruit Salad

Servings: 6 to 8

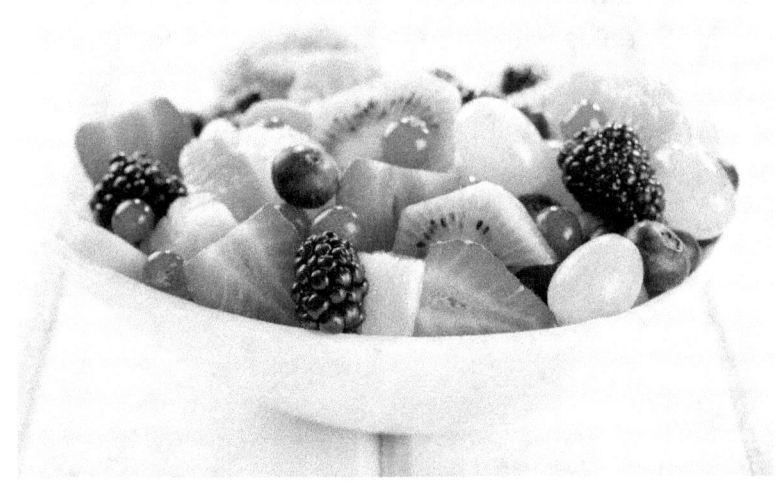

Ingredients:

1 cup fresh blackberries

1 cup green seedless grapes

½ cup fresh blueberries

¼ cup fresh chopped mint

2 cups fresh sliced strawberries

2 fresh limes, halved

2 ripe kiwifruit, peeled and sliced

2 ripe oranges, peeled and chopped

Instructions:

1. In a large bowl, combine all the fruits and toss lightly with the mint.
2. Squeeze the limes over the salad and toss to incorporate.
3. Chill the salad in the refrigerator until ready for serving.

Overnight Raspberry Coconut Oats

Servings: 4

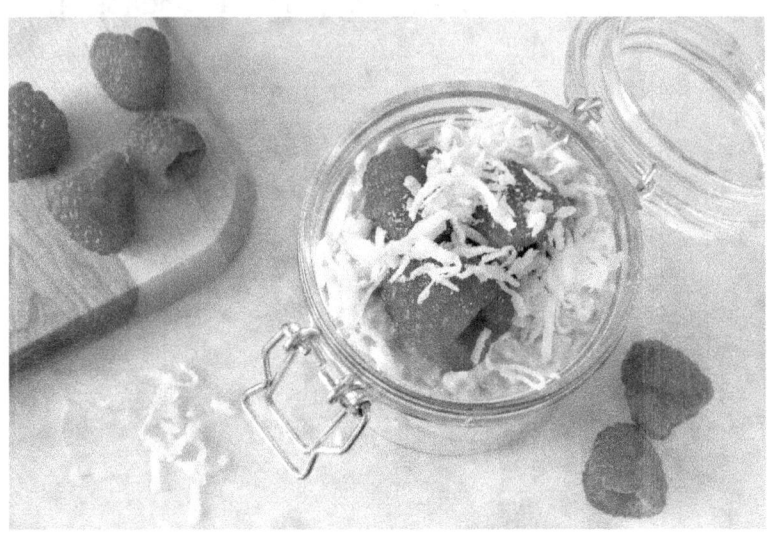

Ingredients:

1 ½ cups old-fashioned oats

1 ½ teaspoon vanilla extract

1 cup fresh raspberries

1 cup skim milk

½ cup shredded unsweetened coconut

2 tablespoons honey or maple syrup

Instructions:

1. In a mixing bowl, add and then stir all of the
   ingredients.

2. Place in a container with a cover. Cover and chill overnight.
3. Serve the oatmeal with raspberries and coconut on top.

Spinach Frittata

Servings: 6 to 8

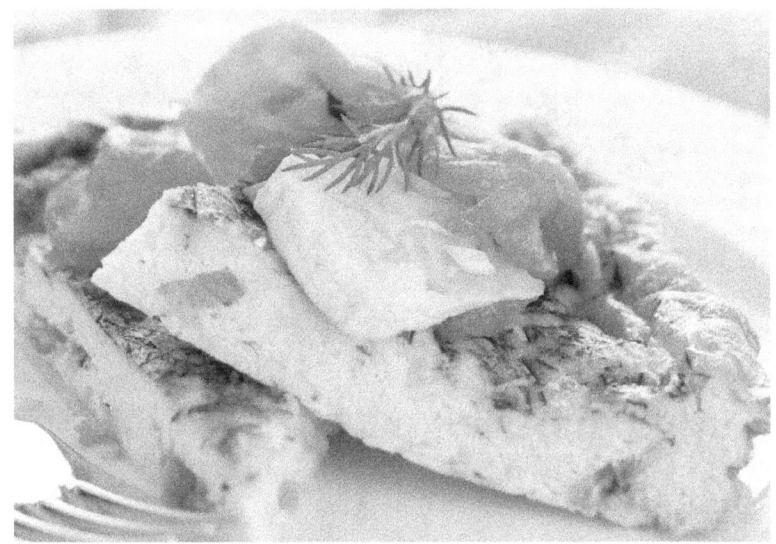

Ingredients:

1 large red pepper, cored and diced

1 large yellow onion, diced

1 tablespoon unsalted butter

¼ cup water

10 large eggs, whisked

2 green onions, sliced thin

Salt and pepper to taste

Instructions:

1. Preheat a broiler to high heat.

2. In a cast iron skillet, melt butter over medium heat.
3. Cook the onion and red pepper in the butter until the onion is translucent.
4. In a bowl, combine the eggs, water, green onion, salt and pepper together and whisk.
5. Add the mixture into the skillet slowly then stir in the spinach.
6. Let the egg cook for about 5 to 6 minutes until almost set then broil for about 2 minutes until the eggs are cooked through.

Apple Chicken Salad

Servings: 6 to 8

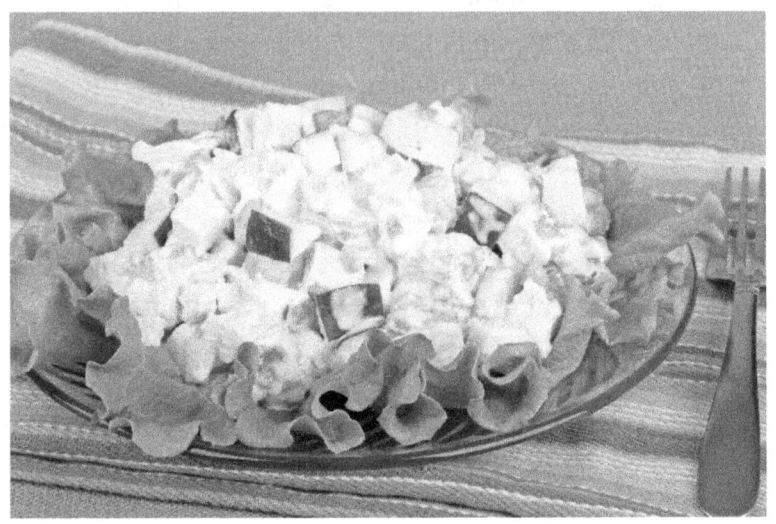

Ingredients:

1 cup seedless grapes, halved

1 tablespoon apple cider vinegar

½ cup diced celery

¼ cup chopped pecans

2 small apples, cored and chopped

¾ cup mayonnaise (made with olive oil)

4 cups cooked chicken breast, chopped

Salt and pepper to taste

Instructions:

1. In a mixing bowl, Whisk the mayonnaise, apple cider vinegar, salt and pepper.
2. Lightly toss to coat the chicken, apple, grapes, celery and pecans in the mixing bowl
3. Sprinkle with salt and pepper to taste.
4. Chill then serve.

Avocado and Mango Salad

Servings: 6

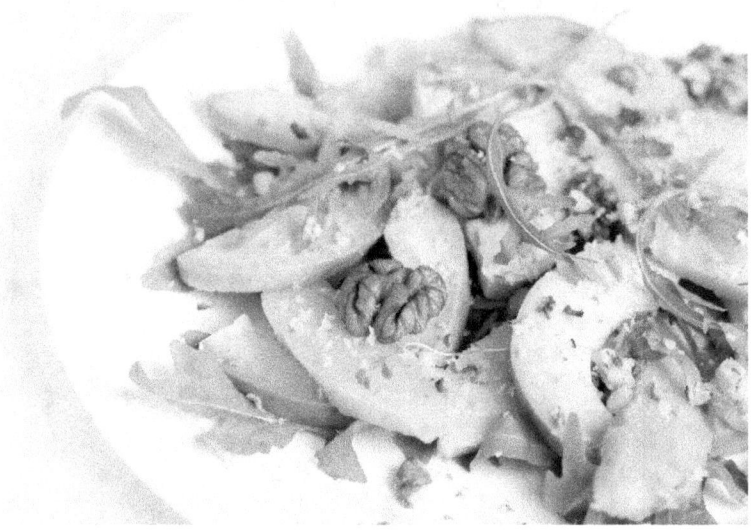

Ingredients:

1 ½ cups sliced mushrooms

1 ripe avocado, pitted and sliced thin

1 ripe mango, pitted and sliced thin

1 tablespoon minced white onion

½ cup sliced green onion

¼ cup extra-virgin olive oil

3 tablespoons red wine vinegar

8 cups fresh spring greens

Pinch dry mustard powder

Instructions:

1. In a mixing bowl, lightly toss the spring greens, mushrooms and green onion.
2. In another bowl, whisk the rest of the ingredients and toss in with the salad when about to serve.

Egg Salad and Chives

Servings: 6 to 8

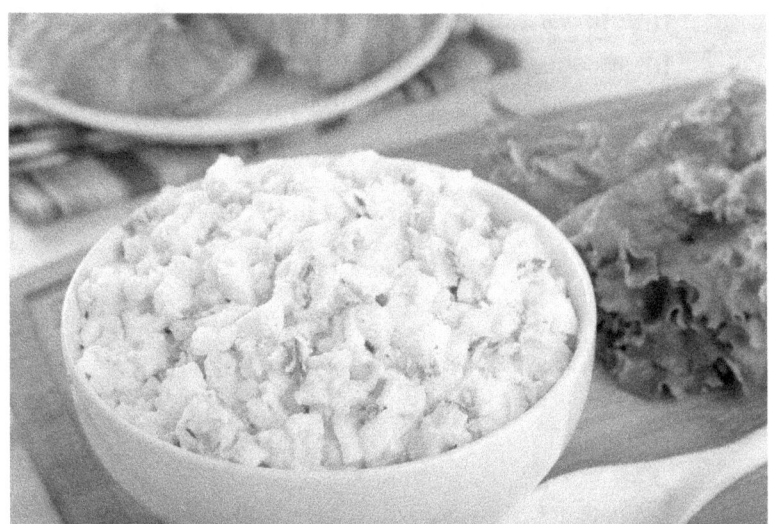

Ingredients:

1 ½ tablespoons Dijon mustard

1/3 cup diced red onion

12 large hardboiled eggs, peeled and chopped

2 stalks celery, diced

3 tablespoons chopped chives

¾ cup mayonnaise

Salt and pepper to taste

Instructions:

1. In a mixing bowl, whisk the mayonnaise, mustard, salt and pepper.

2. Lightly toss in the eggs, celery, onion and chives.
3. Sprinkle some salt and pepper to taste.
4. Chill before serving.

Strawberry Spinach Salad with Balsamic

Servings: 6

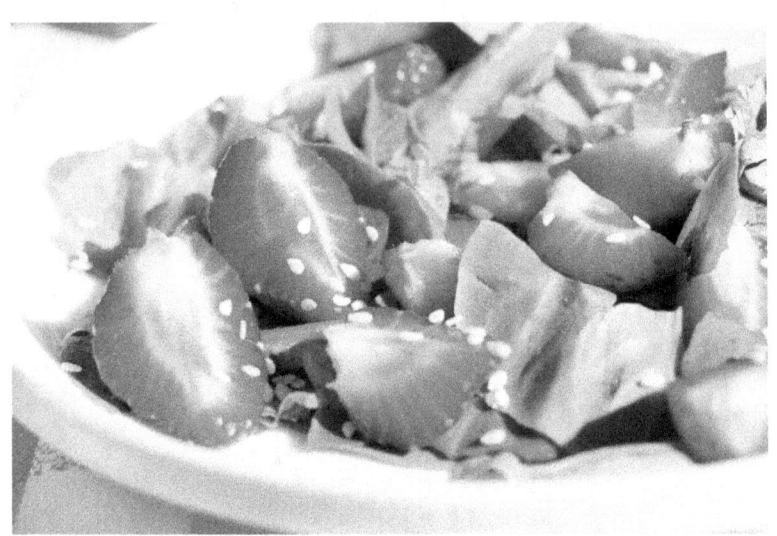

Ingredients:

8 cups fresh baby spinach

1 ½ cups sliced mushrooms

½ small red onion, sliced thin

1 ¾ cups diced strawberries, divided

3 tablespoons olive oil

3 tablespoons balsamic vinegar

Pinch salt and pepper

Instructions:

1. In a bowl, lightly toss the spinach with mushrooms, red onion and 1 ½ cups diced strawberries.
2. Divide the salad into plates and sprinkle some sesame seeds on top.
3. In a food processor, add the rest of the ingredients and blend until the mixture is smooth. Use as a dressing.
4. Serve.

Smooth Curry Vegetable Soup

Servings: 6 to 8

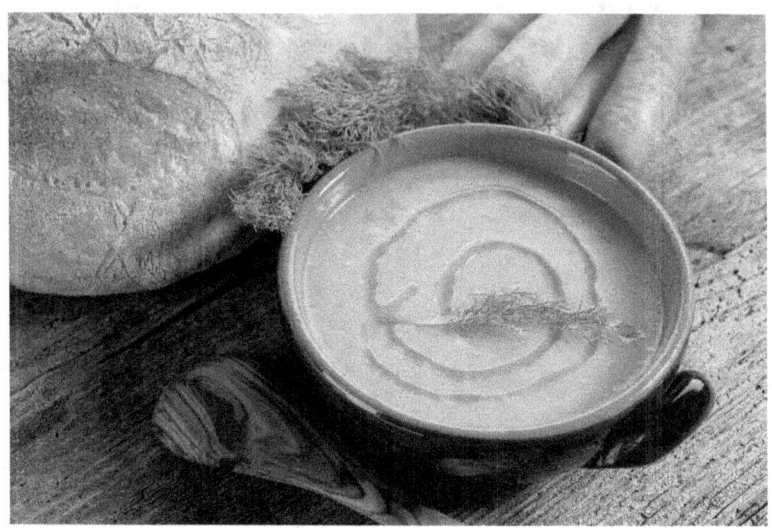

Ingredients:

1 large sweet potato, peeled and chopped

1 lbs. baby carrots, chopped or sliced

1 small yellow onion, chopped

1 tablespoon lemon juice

1 tablespoon minced garlic

1 tablespoon olive oil

1 teaspoon curry powder

5 cups chicken or vegetable broth

Salt and pepper to taste

Instructions:

1. In a large saucepan, heat the oil over medium heat.
2. Cook the carrots, sweet potato, onion and garlic until the onion is translucent.
3. Add the rest of the ingredients and then let it boil.
4. Once boiling, reduce to a simmer until the vegetables are cooked and tender.
5. Remove from heat and using an immersion blender, puree until smooth.
6. Add salt and pepper to taste.
7. Place in bowls and serve hot.

Spiced Pumpkin Soup

Servings: 8 to 10

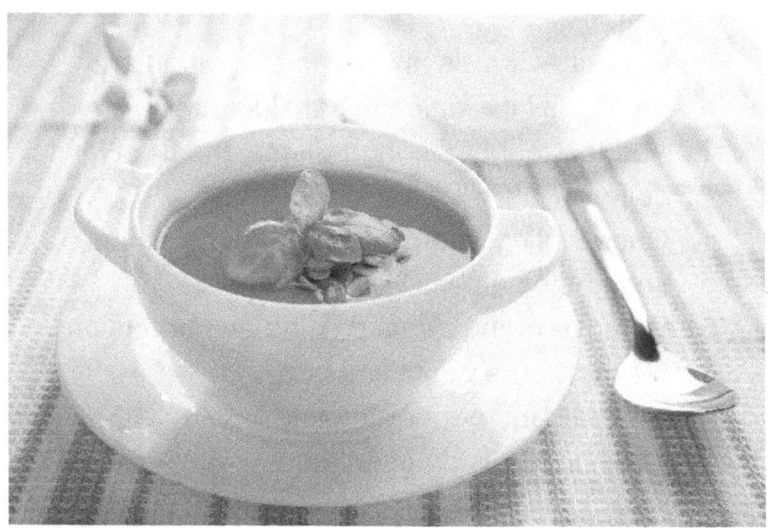

Ingredients:

1 ½ cups chicken broth or vegetable broth

1 cup heavy cream

1 large sweet onion, chopped

1 tablespoon olive oil

1 teaspoon ground cinnamon

2 (15-ounce) cans pureed pumpkin

2 cloves minced garlic

4 cups water

Salt and pepper to taste

Instructions:

1. In a large saucepan, heat the oil in medium heat.
2. Cook the onion and garlic until the onion is translucent.
3. Stir in the rest of the ingredients then boil.
4. Reduce to a simmer and simmer until the pumpkin is tender.
5. Remove the pan from the heat.
6. Using an immersion blender, puree the soup and veggies until smooth.
7. Add salt and pepper to taste.
8. Enjoy hot.

Roasted Acorn Squash Soup

Servings: 6 to 8

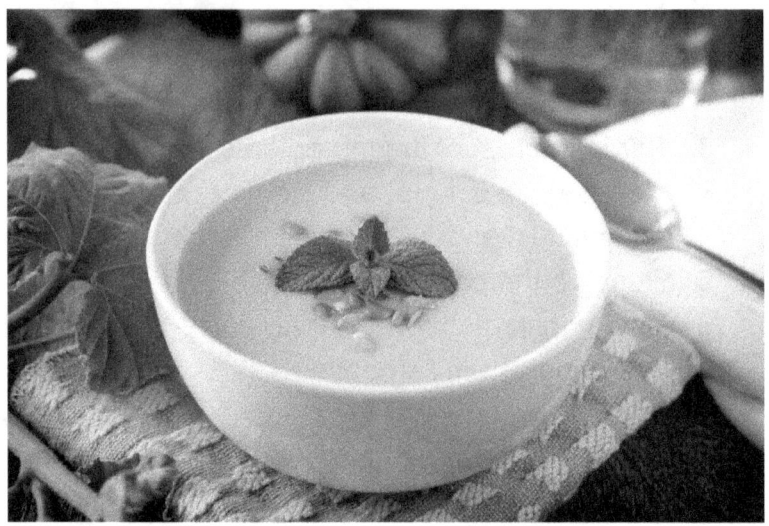

Ingredients:

1 stalk celery, diced

1 sweet onion, chopped

1 tablespoon minced garlic

1 teaspoon dried thyme

2 medium carrots, peeled and chopped

2 to 3 tablespoons olive oil

3 medium acorn squash

5 cups chicken or vegetable broth

Salt and pepper to taste

Instructions:

1. Turn on your oven and preheat to 350°F/275°C.
2. Cut the squash required in half lengthwise and remove the seeds.
3. Cost the squash halves with olive oil and place on a rimmed baking dish.
4. Sprinkle with salt and pepper then bake for about 30 to 45 minutes or until the squash is tender all the way through.
5. Cool the squash before handling then scoop out the flesh into a clean bowl.
6. In a large saucepan, heat the oil over medium heat.
7. Cook the carrot, celery, onion and garlic until the onion is translucent.
8. Add and stir the rest of the ingredients in the saucepan and boil.
9. Once boiling, reduce to a simmer and simmer until the vegetables are tender.
10. Remove from heat once tender. Using an immersion blender, puree until smooth.
11. Sprinkle with salt and pepper to taste.
12. Serve hot.

Balsamic Grilled Salmon

Servings: 6

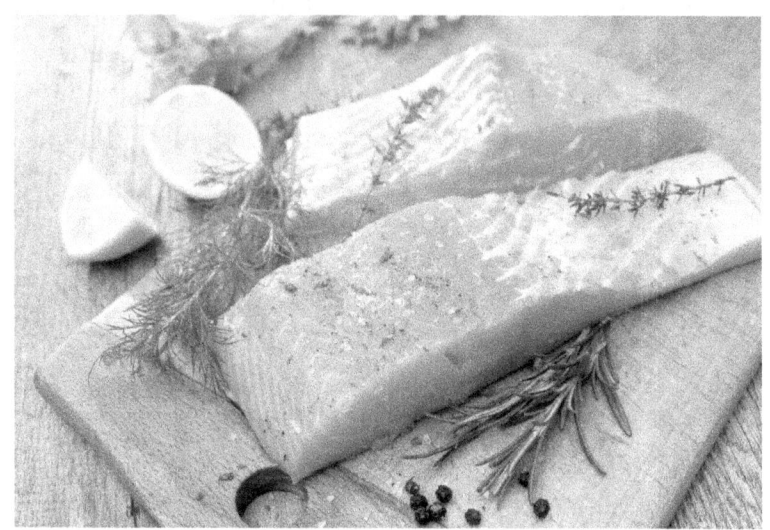

Ingredients:

1 to 2 tablespoon olive oil

1/3 cup balsamic vinegar

1/3 cup dry white wine

2 tablespoons maple syrup

3 tablespoons fresh lemon juice

6 (6-ounce) boneless salmon fillets

Salt and pepper to taste

Instructions:

1. In a saucepan, add in balsamic vinegar, wine, lemon juice and maple syrup over low to medium heat.
2. Simmer and cook until thickened, about 12 t o15 minutes then set aside.
3. Brush the grates of your grill with olive oil and preheat to high.
4. Season the salmon with salt and pepper and brush with oil.
5. Cook the fillets in your grill for about 5 minutes on each side.
6. Serve with the glaze.

Skillet Steaks

Servings: 6

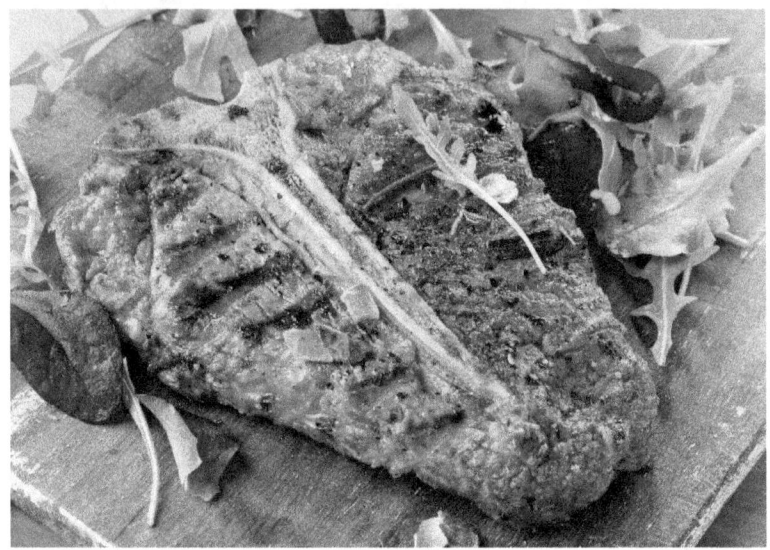

Ingredients:

1 tablespoon coconut oil

1 tablespoon minced garlic

2 (10 to 12-ounce) New York strip steaks

2 tablespoons unsalted butter

Salt and pepper to taste

Instructions:

1. The steaks should be at room temperature when cooking.
2. In a large cast iron skillet, heat oil over high heat.

3. Season the steaks with salt and pepper to taste.
4. Place the steaks on the skillet and flash fry for about 3 minutes on each side until browned.
5. When the steaks are done, lower the heat to low to medium and melt the butter.
6. Baste the steak with the butter for about 1 to 2 minutes and remove from the pan and transfer to a cutting board.
7. Place in a serving plate with foil and let it rest for 10 minutes before serving.

Healthy Meatloaf

Servings: 6 to 8

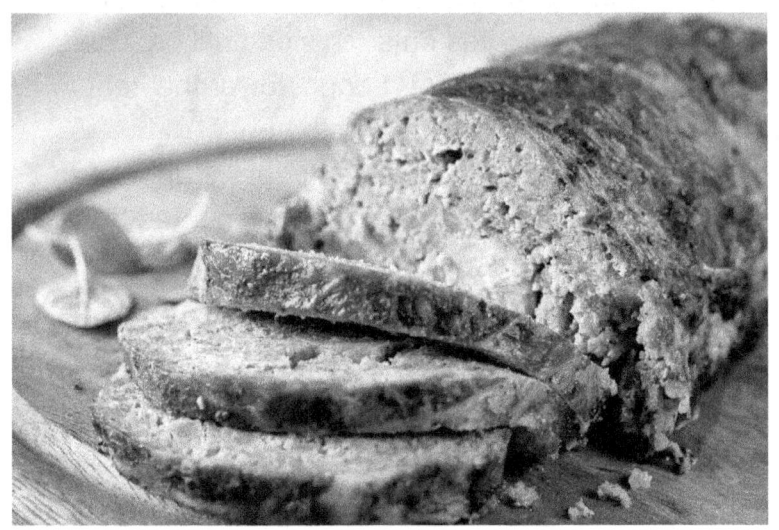

Ingredients:

1 lbs. lean ground beef

1 tablespoon Dijon mustard

½ lbs. lean ground lamb

¼ cup tomato sauce

¼ lbs. lean ground pork

2 large eggs, beaten

2 tablespoons Worcestershire sauce

2/3 cup whole-wheat flour

Salt and pepper to taste

Instructions:

1. Grease a bread pan with some butter or oil and preheat your oven to 400°F/200°C.
2. In a mixing bowl, stir the ingredients together. Spread around the pan evenly, pressed.
3. Let it bake for about 50 to 60 minute until the internal temperature is 165°F/75°C.
4. Turn the pan over and transfer the meatloaf on a cutting board. Let it rest for 10 minutes before cutting and serving.

Grilled Salmon with Coconut Mango Sauce

Servings: 6

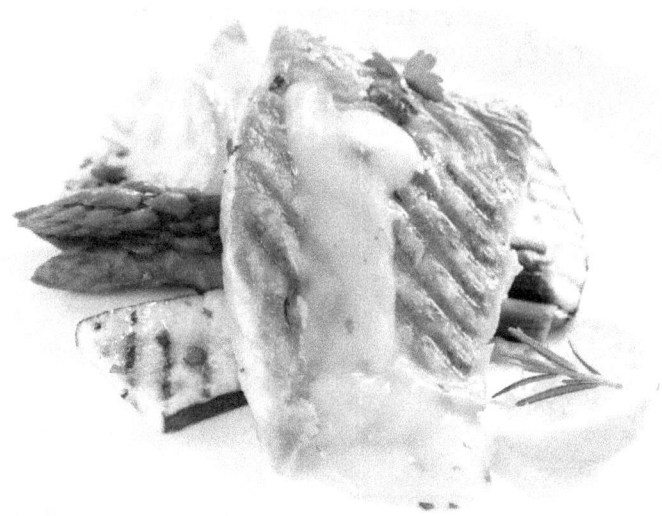

Ingredients:

1 ½ ripe mango, pitted and chopped

1 to 2 tablespoons olive oil, or as needed

½ bunch fresh cilantro

½ cup canned coconut milk

6 (6-ounce) boneless salmon fillets

Salt and pepper to taste

Instructions:

1. Brush the grates of the grill with oil and preheat the grill to high heat.
2. Season the salmon with salt and pepper and brush with some oil.
3. Grill the fillets for about 5 minutes on each side depending on the thickness of the salmon. It is finished cooking when the meat flakes easily.
4. In a blender, add the rest of the ingredients and blend until smooth.
5. When the salmon is done cooking, serve with the sauce.

Easy Chocolate Froyo

Servings: 8 to 10

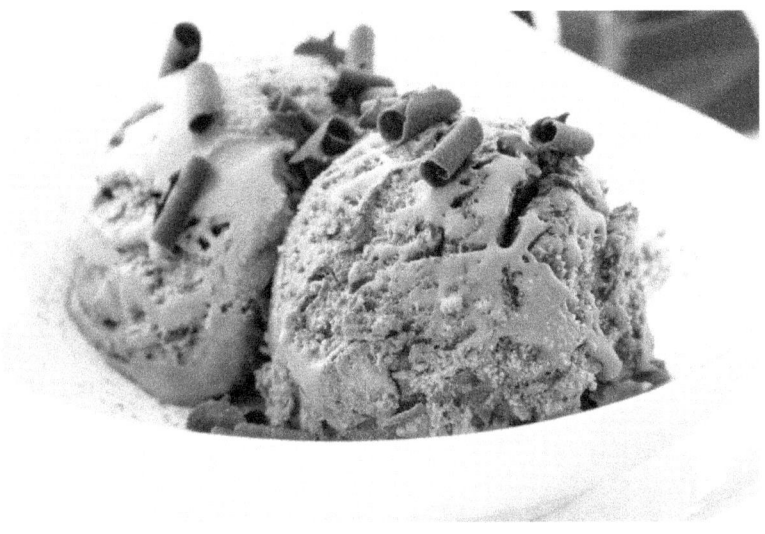

Ingredients:

1 cup mini chocolate chips

1 tablespoon cornstarch

1 tablespoon vanilla extract

1 to 1 ½ teaspoons liquid Stevia

¼ cup unsweetened cocoa powder

2 ½ cups plain Greek yogurt

2 cups heavy cream

4 large egg yolks, whisked

Instructions:

1. In a mixing bowl, beat the yogurt and cream until soft peaks form.
2. Whisk in the egg yolks, vanilla extract and cocoa powder.
3. Add the stevia and cornstarch and whisk until combines and then fold in the chocolate chips carefully.
4. Using an ice cream maker, pour the mixture and freeze according to the manufacturer's instructions.

Vanilla Bean Frozen Yogurt

Servings: 8 to 10

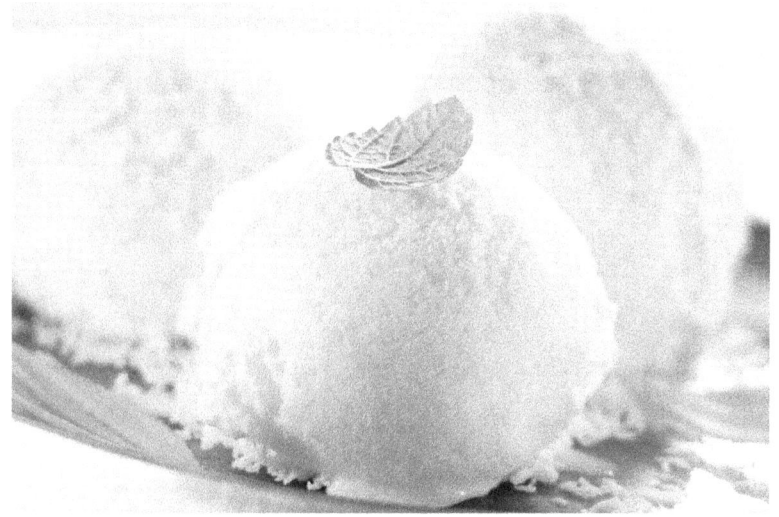

Ingredients:

1 tablespoon cornstarch

1 teaspoon liquid Stevia

2 ½ cups vanilla Greek yogurt

2 cups heavy cream

2 fresh vanilla beans, halved

2 tablespoons vanilla extract

4 large egg yolks, whisked

Instructions:

1. In a mixing bowl, beat the yogurt and cream until soft peaks form.

2. Add in the egg yolks, vanilla extract and scrape the vanilla bean and mix.
3. Add the stevia and cornstarch and mix well.
4. Using an ice cream maker, pour the mixture and freeze according to the manufacturer's instructions.

Chia Seed Pudding

Servings: 6

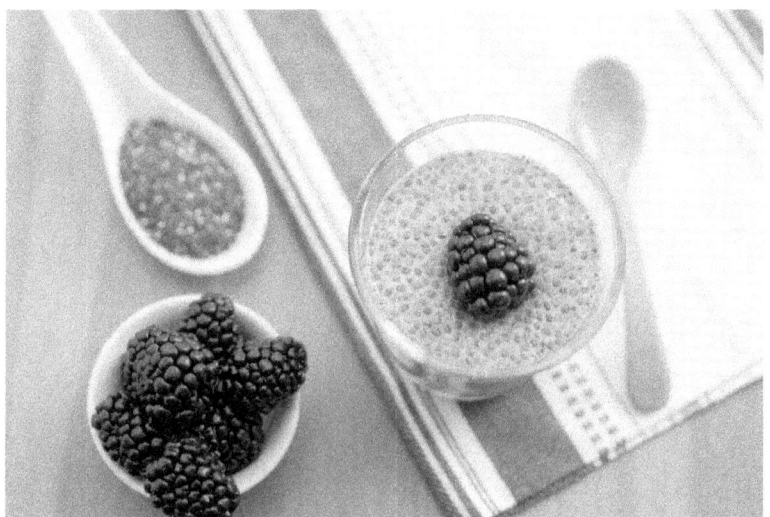

Ingredients:

1 ½ cups heavy cream

1 ¼ cups chia seeds

1 teaspoon liquid Stevia

1/3 cup unsweetened cocoa powder

2 ½ cups skim milk

Instructions:

1. In a blender, add all of the ingredients.
2. Blend until smooth, about 30 to 60 seconds.
3. Spoon into dessert cups or container.
4. Chill for at least 20 minutes before serving.

Creamy Avocado-Based Chocolate Mousse

Servings: 4 to 6

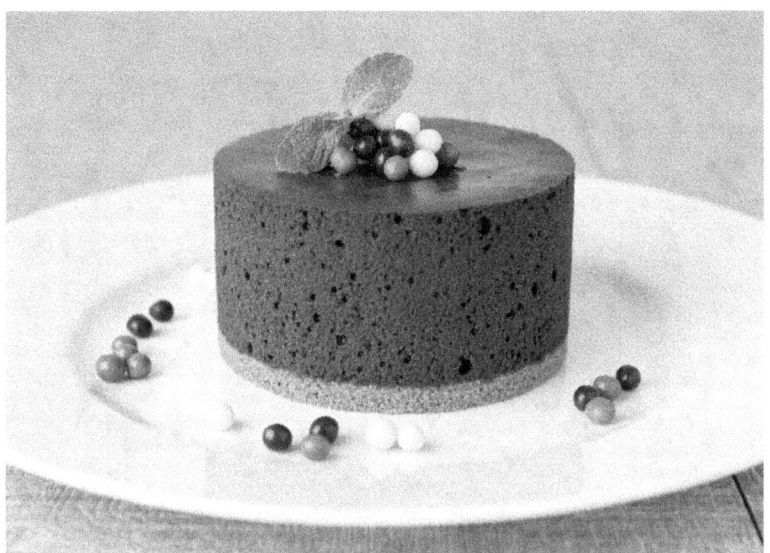

Ingredients:

1 ½ teaspoon vanilla extract

½ cup heavy cream

¼ cup raw honey

¼ cup unsweetened cocoa powder

2 large ripe avocado, pitted and chopped

Instructions:

1. In a blender, add all of the ingredients.
2. Blend until smooth, about 30 to 60 seconds.
3. Scoop the mousse into dessert cups.
4. Chill for at least 20 minutes before serving.

Conclusion

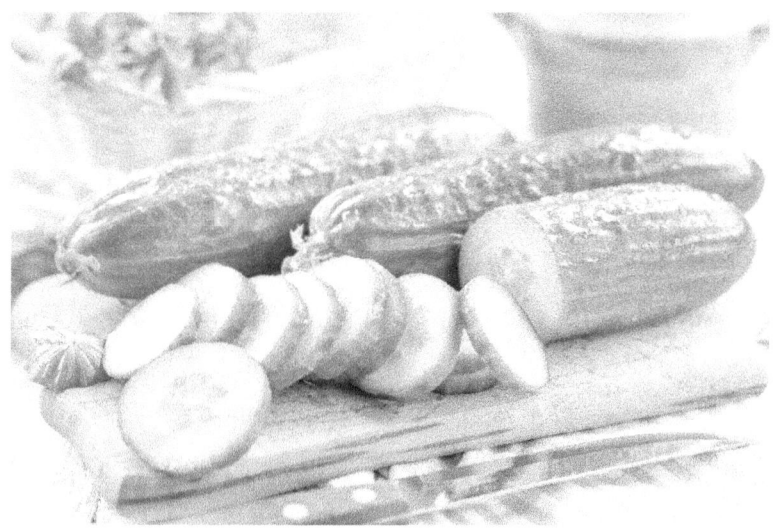

It may be difficult to make changes in your diet, but with these yummy recipes, I won't be as difficult. By eating the recipes in this book or looking for healthy recipes, you can easily shed off years on your appearance. Looking and feeling younger doesn't need plastic surgery, it just needs a good anti-aging diet foundation and you can start this today! This book will be your perfect start to a younger you. Pick out a recipe and try it out.